YOU
LOSE WEIGHT WITHOUT GOING ON DIET!

CW00495105

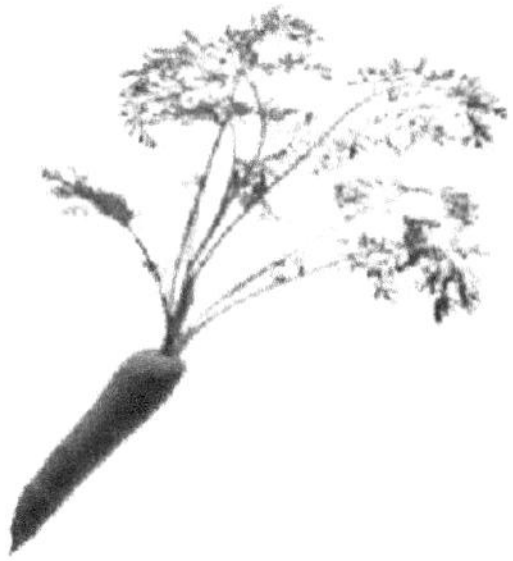

TIARNA COMBS

© **Copyright** – Tiarna Combs

2022 All rights reserved

This book or parts thereof may not be reproduced in any form, stored in any retrieval system, or transmitted in any form by any means—electronic, mechanical, photocopy, recording, or otherwise—without prior written permission of the publisher. All rights reserved.

Disclaimer: The information contained within this eBook is given solely by the authors own adhered to knowledge and thorough researched of said subject. The contents herein have been made as accurate, and up to date, with reliable information as possible. Readers, please acknowledge these are the authors researched and studied subjects and is not engaging/supporting in any legal, medical, or financial Advice. If at all concerned to any medical, or fitness regime please refer to your own medical practitioner guidance.

ISBN: 978-1-7391038-7-3

TC Publications

Table Of Contents

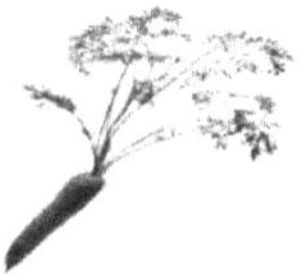

Our Fast-Paced Lifestyle

With our Fast-paced lifestyle we live in today it is having a huge and sometimes detrimental effect on our health and mental well-being.

Obesity and Mental Health problems have reached epic proportions. The pace of life has just got faster and faster and sometimes we struggle to keep up!

This often and can result in stress related illnesses of all kinds because we just cannot keep up the pace!

To help us cope with this stress were turning to food to use as a prop maybe to comfort us or to try to combat our 'stress' some professionals call this 'comfort eating'. Problem is with this extra 'comfort eating' were piling on the pounds like never before and in turn it is resulting in Obesity epidemics.

Obesity is not only present in America, but it is here in the UK and the problem is getting worse, younger children are getting Obesity problems like never!

The sad realisation is that the young and teens are storing up health problems for when they are older!
Add to our woes were seeing a huge rise in mental health problems that are related to our lifestyles, sometimes it can seem like a vicious circle a circle that needs to be broken!

We cannot change the pace of life it is with us forever!
After all it is not our fault everything has changed everything today is at breakneck speed! from times gone by……
but we can adjust our lifestyles to keep up and try to compliment with it! It really does not have to be this way!

This guide-book is written not to judge or moralise but to guide you point you in the right direction.

Help you keep up with modern life and the pace, show you with some pointers to change your health and your life for the better!

It's not a Diet Book its mainly an advice or guidance book to help you stop making the same mistakes in regard to food, diet, and your wellbeing.

CHAPTER 1

How Can we Change Our Life for the Better?

Our pace of life yes has quickened and with this fast pace our lifestyles have become increasingly sedentary. With technology taking us over after all everything and most things conducted with technology today! For example, we sit at our desks in our office-based jobs!

We can spend 8 or 9 hours at the office daily we come home to relax or unwind only to spend another 4 or 5 hours slumped in front of the TV (we feel too tired to do anything else) what with the daily commute too!

Plus being stuck in our cars because of traffic jams! And getting stressed and frustrated trying to reach our destination!

So, we slump ourselves in front of the TV to relax we then go to bed and do the same thing over again next day! We need to change or adjust!
Technology has also taken over our children too!

Children are on their laptops or tablets, game boy's consoles, etc they're sadly not as active as previous generations who used to regularly play outside after school and keeping active, instead they're being more sedentary and playing on their 'Technology games instead!
Not realising the harm sedentary lifestyle is doing it is influencing us all!
Is it any wonder then we have a growing obesity epidemic here in UK and in other cities worldwide!

Ask yourself do you wish you were healthier, have more energy, be fitter and achieve more out of life?
It really does not have to be this way!

- Diabetes
- Heart Disease
- Osteoporosis
- Obesity
- High Blood Pressure
- Arthritis
- Stress
- Anxiety
- Depression
- Dementia

Scary isn't it!
Above are just some of the conditions that many are afflicted with and which our hospitals are treating daily in this modern fast paced lifestyle were all a part of and having to live with.

I say having to because there is no escape, modern times have just got faster & faster over the years and it's affecting our health like never before!

We keep piling on the weight and our health is suffering our bodies rebel by giving us all manner of horrible symptoms which can invariably lead to any of the above conditions and more ......
The list goes on ......

We need to try to change and do things differently but how can we when were all part of the same system same lifestyle?
We cannot change the fast pace of life but we can try to make some changes for ourselves, try to change some of our behaviours and try to encourage our children too!

The title of this book says it all, but it's not just about losing weight it's about how we manage our bodies mentally and physically if you persevere 'You can change your life around.
By doing other things and looking after ourselves.

One thing we will not be going on a 'diet' keep that in mind, you're just changing some things in your life for the better keep that change for the rest of your life!

This will be your daily Mantra.

'My life is a product of My actions for the Better!'

There are Four basic solutions we can use to start our brand-new journey:

- Be Creative: Change our Diet, Change our Recipes, Change our Food.
- Be Aware: Aware of everything we Eat Consciously and **Unconsciously**
- Learn how to Relax: By learning how to really relax ourselves we are Keeping Stress at bay
- Fitness: Keep us MOVING or AIM TO get ourselves fitter!
- SLEEP: Make sure you make time for It.

These are our goals to start with:

If we can stick with our new schedule, we will over time begin to see subtle changes to our health. We'll start to feel a brand-new outlook, and we're learning to keep up with the fast pace of life.

Summary:

To adjust to our modern fast paced lifestyle, we need to:

- Change our old ways of doing things
- Aim to get back our fitness (at our own pace)
- Change our eating habits (more healthy food options)
- Experiment with new eating habits
- Learn to relax more*make time to relax
- Get more sleep *make time to get more sleep
- Discipline ourselves for change
- Show determination* even if things don't go to plan try again next day
- Not giving up

CHAPTER 2

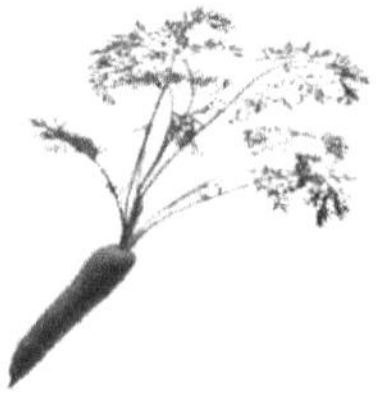

Breaking the unhealthy eating Cycle

To begin we are going to be changing some things in our lives. Eating sensible foods, eating less calorific foods, cutting out or curbing junk foods, sugar laden foods.

The long-term solution for weight loss is to be creative and change our eating habits!

Many people resort to quirky diets there have over the years been many out their! Pineapple Diet, Carrot Diet, Atkins Diet, Beverley Hills Hollywood Style Diet, liquid Only diet the list goes on.

Some of these diets have been shown to work! And can shed pounds rapidly but at what cost health wise? And when you have got bored with the bland variety offered you give up only to pile the weight back on a couple of weeks later!
Also, some fad diets leave you feeling hungry, irritable, and deprived so you give up and start unhealthy eating again!

For our first discipline we are going to examine how best we can eat food which is healthy, looks good and appetizing leaving us feeling nourished without feeling guilty.
Help us to lose weight healthily whilst still feeling energised, being happy with ourselves, and no pressure!

We shall examine the best foods to consume without 'going on a Diet' and starving ourselves! We are basically looking after ourselves at the same time as watching what we are eating!

To reiterate our aim is to eat healthy foods and to lose weight gradually over time- no rush just our first discipline to change our lifestyle regarding our food intake and the type of foods were consuming!

So, to Adjust to our modern fast paced lifestyle get fit and healthy and help get you to where you want to be on your part it will take some effort and change and some discipline.

Firstly, we need to create new eating habits and adjusting our diet to healthier foods.
Before we go onto the next chapter, I want to give you some extra tips on food intake.
Did you know that one pound of Fat is equal to
3.500 calories!

I know were not going on a Diet! This is Not a Diet book! But keeping with our 'New You' outlook and again changing some things.

If you can aim to reach a goal of cutting out say 300-500 Empty Calories a day from your diet and combine with (later on) some light exercise to start you can easily lose about 1 pound a week! Imagine that!

You don't have to start with 500max calories to lose you can adjust to say 100-200 loss of empty calories a day from your usual daily diet for it to make a difference!

And as you notice the difference this will spur you on to want to aim for more gradually aiming for 500 empty calorie a day loss!

Just do want you feel comfortable with it isn't a race with anyone it's just for you!

We're going to be eating healthily but at the same time cutting out those Empty Calories!

Those tempting ones that might look good but in the long term do more harm!

E.g., sugary sweets, calorie laden desserts, sugary unhealthy cakes, sugar laden cereals, sugary laden fruit juices, sugar laden milk shakes, etc...... the list goes on!

Later on in this book I will give you a table of the good and the bad foods you can add to your daily diary you're going to be keeping.

This is where you'll be well ahead and well aware you will see beforehand where you keep going wrong in relation to those tempting but hidden calories!
We still need some carbohydrates in our diet as they are a source of fuel for the body.

Saying that there are good carbs and bad carbs.
Bad carbs include white bread, cookies, candies, and cereals loaded with sugar.

These bad carbs contribute to your weight gain and if you continue eating these bad foods it can raise the risk of heart disease or type 2 diabetes, try to switch to healthy whole grains to protect you from these health conditions.
I have included a table of Good Carbs and the Bad Carbs for you to keep and for you to be aware of in your new healthy living course.

CHAPTER 3

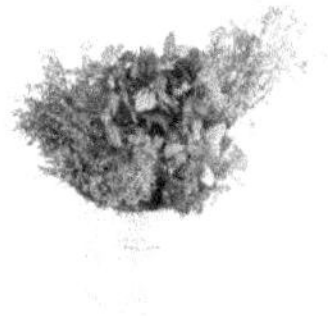

What Healthier Foods then can we eat?

Do you Know you can eat pies, cottage pies, chilli con carne, spaghetti Bolognese, tuna pasta, Lasagne etc….

without adding Meat. All these foods and dishes can be prepared without containing any animal products at all. Have you heard of:

- Soya?
- Or Quinoa?
- Tofu?
- Seitan/Wheat Protein?
- Quorn?
- Tempeh?
- Green Spelt?

- Textured Vegetable Protein?
- Amaranth?
- Whole grain millet?
- Wild Rice?

I'll go through a brief informative description on each of these great protein rich foods, meat alternatives. They are healthy, good for you, low in fat, very versatile and not a meat product or animal ingredient amongst them!

Soya:

What is Soya? Is it good for me? Soya Beans are very high in Protein contain a good source vitamin, minerals, also isoflavones, with also beneficial plant compounds.

Some studies have suggested soya can alleviate symptoms of menopause, and reduce your risk of breast cancer, and prostate cancer.

Soya protein has also been known to lower the body's
natural LDL cholesterol producing capacity in the Liver (Source info*BDA UK dietitians) Fermented and unfermented Soya have a high range of essential amino acids which are similar to animal protein.

There are a variety of Soya products on the market today and these can include Soya burgers and Soya Sausages Soya mince / chunks (textured vegetable protein)

Quinoa: Quinoa (pronounced ke-NO-ah)

Quinoa is high in fibre, protein and has a low glycaemic index. These properties have all been linked to weight loss and improved health.

This 'superfood" is very popular amongst the health conscious and you can see why, it is packed with Protein, Vitamins and minerals, Fibre, and is gluten-free and been recommended for people on a gluten-free diet.

Quinoa is often used as a substitute for rice. But can be used for other healthy dishes too.

Quinoa has a slightly nutty taste, when cooked and gives a soft and fluffy appearance.

It can also be made into flour, flakes and various foods like pasta and bread, according to the (grains and nutrition council*)

Quinoa originates from Peru, and grows in Chile and Bolivia (**Quinoa** means 'mother grain' in the Incan language

Tofu: Is an excellent source of Protein it is derived from Soya it is made from soybeans which are curdled and pressed and made into blocks similar to making cheese. This rich source of protein which contains nine essential amino acids, a whole host of minerals and iron, calcium and vitamin B1 you can see why it has become more and more popular!

It too like soya has also been known to lower the body's natural **LDL cholesterol.**

Tofu like Soya contains isoflavones which are similar to the female oestrogen so therefore, mimics the action of oestrogen thus with the same properties of soya can alleviate distressing symptoms of menopause and can help to reduce your risk of breast cancer, menopause and can help to reduce your risk of breast cancer, this is why more and more women are including soya-rich foods into their daily diet.

Seitan/Wheat Protein:

Seitan (pronounced SAY-tan) is a type of Wheat Protein.

It is also called gluten, wheat protein, or wheat gluten. and textured wheat protein

Seitan is a meat-free alternative with a texture that resembles animal- based meat.

Seitan is a very popular staple for vegans and use this ingredient in their diets and recipes.

This Seitan/Wheat Protein is known for its health-giving benefits:

Cholesterol-Free Contains lots of B vitamins and Minerals plus iron. High in Proteins and Low in calories Plant based Protein.

How can I use **Seitan**?

Basically, you can use Seitan as you would normally use meat,

in casseroles, chilli dishes, or homemade pies, even in a stir fry, or make up your usual sandwich but without the meat!

Quorn: Is a type of protein-rich food made from an edible fungus and used as a meat substitute. Another name for Quorn is its ingredient Mycoprotein

Quorn is sold as a meat substitute and works well for a cooking ingredient.

You can also purchase a wide range of Quorn products

e.g., sausages, pies, lasagnes and ready-made meals as it has become very popular for vegans and vegetarians and anyone who does not eat meat.

Chia Seeds: Chia seeds contain large amounts of Fibre and omega-3 fatty acids, plenty of high-quality Protein, and several essential minerals iron, calcium, magnesium and antioxidants. They may improve digestive health, blood levels of heart-healthy omega-3s.

You can eat **Chia seeds** raw or prepared in dishes. Also, can be sprinkled on salads, cereal, yogurt and vegetables. You can even add them to your favourite sandwich.

Tempeh: Tempeh is a high protein food made from Soya beans it has its origins in Indonesia it is a great substitute for Meat in Vegan and Vegetarian dishes. The way to cook Tempeh is very similar to tofu. It can be added into soups, chilli con-carne, casseroles, Pies, you can even grate it or try adding it to a stir fry.
Many recipes recommend softening the tempeh before you cook with it or add it to a dish for best results is follow pack instructions for preparation of dishes.

Where to buy: **Tempeh** can be purchased in most health food stores and some large Supermarket stores.

Green Spelt: Green Spelt is a wholegrain and an alternative to rice it is called green spelt because it has been harvested earlier when it is still green.

It is also a form of wheat.

It can be used in place of boiled rice or risotto rice, can also make a nice salad dish. There are varieties of spelt to use which can be used in the same way high in protein and low in fat.

Textured Vegetable Protein:

Textured or texturized vegetable protein, also known as textured soy protein, soy meat, or soya chunks is a defatted soy flour product, a by-product of extracting soybean oil.

It is often used as a meat analogue or meat extender.

It is quick to cook, with a protein content comparable to certain meats. (Source info *Wikipedia)

TVP can be used or added to any type of dish similar soya it can be added in place of meat for dishes such as chilli con -carne, cottage pies, spaghetti Bolognese, it is a meat substitute made from soybeans, high in protein, low in fat, it is common in veggie burgers and vegetarian dishes.

You can purchase flavoured **TVP** and unflavoured, it is very popular with vegans and vegetarians. Or anyone who does not eat meat.
There are a lot of new products now coming on the market and it is accelerating rapidly especially in America and in UK for people who do not want to eat animal meat anymore, who are now choosing more healthier options for themselves and for the good of the Planet.

Amaranth: Amaranth is a wheat grain its properties are high in calcium, magnesium, iron, phosphorous and potassium, and the only grain to contain large amounts of vitamin C.
It has anti-inflammatory and cancer-preventive properties.

Amaranth It is high in protein also been known to benefit heart health, and contains a rich source of phytosterols

Whole Grain Millet: This Grain is registered by the whole grains council for being the world's most important grain.

Several varieties have been recorded of this millet grain such as foxtail, finger, kodo, pearl, and little millets.

These grains are all free of gluten and very high in antioxidants, and Foxtail millet has been shown in a study to reduce triglyceride levels and increase good cholesterol.

Wild Rice: Wild Rice again is a whole grain which include the bran, germ, and endosperm.

Has a powerhouse full of protein this grain also has a delicious nutty flavour. This wild rice is excellent for people who have gluten or wheat sensitivities, or who suffer from celiac disease.

Wild Rice is an excellent source of many minerals such as **magnesium, vitamin b6, zinc, niacin, manganese, plus is loaded with Fibre.**

If you consumed wild rice every day it will improve your heart health and study shown reduce the risk of type 2 diabetes.

How To Add More Whole Grains Into Your Diet

- Invest in a healthy breakfast by adding whole-grain cereals
- like Oats or bran flakes
- Whole Grain Bread or Seeded Bread is so much healthier than white bread for sandwiches
- For meals or dishes substitute white rice and choose brown rice, quinoa or wild rice.

- For recipes or dishes substitute breadcrumbs for rolled oats or crushed whole-wheat bran
- In soups or stews add wild rice or barley to get extra vitamins

CHAPTER 4

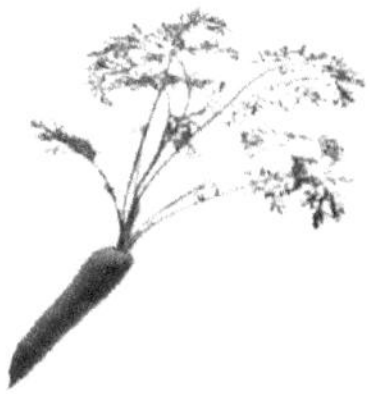

Weight Loss Tips to Take Note for your Journey.

If your goal is permanent weight loss your key to success is Not to Diet

Focus instead on several things you can easily do every day.

First Rule: Don't beat yourself up on Targets! Just set yourself a realistic goal; if you find that your goal was missed just start again don't beat yourself up.

With my Tips I'll be giving you if you try to follow them and put into practice this could help you in your weight loss goals and you could easily lose one to two pounds a week without too much effort!

Our first goal is to make changes to our eating habits, and later on in the chapter I want to introduce you to keeping active with some light exercises to start) I will explain more in regard to exercise in another chapter!
Nothing too strenuous for a beginner I want to show you how to get moving more!

Now to our Daily Tips: Below I've added a list of your daily tips to try to stick with don't worry if you can't on some days stick with it but try to add some of the tips into your daily lifestyle

Your Daily Routine Tips:

Tip 1: Try to eat Breakfast Every Day!

Try to eat breakfast every day! There is a myth If I skip breakfast that will help my weight loss!
Wrong by not eating breakfast it can lead to more calorie gain because you'll feel hungry half way through the morning grab something unhealthy to give you a boost for more energy, which is probably laden with sugar, or full of the wrong calories or empty calories and you'll eat more of it by trying to keep your energy levels going.

Thus, will gain the wrong type of weight being **'Fat storage weight'** which is a lot harder to shift or lose!
Studies show people who eat breakfast (healthy food) breakfast have lower **BMI's.**
(Body mass index) than people who skip breakfast and perform tasks better whether at work or School/college.

The type of breakfasts to keep you energised are **'Whole grain Cereals'** or low-fat **low sugar** cereals, (I will list some healthy sample breakfasts for you to try! At the end of this chapter)

Tip 2: Avoid Heavy Sauces

Try to avoid heavy sauces e.g., those laden with full fat and sugar ingredients in them check the ingredients.
Back and front of packets or do some research what is in the product.
Not just on Sauce packs check any foods the front labels for fats and sugar content; also, the colour system red symbol is always a bad food choice as it signifies high sugars or fats!

Tip 3: Make Yourself Variety Interesting Meals but Healthy Too

Eat foods you enjoy eating not boring and bland! Yes, they need to be healthy too but also fulfilling and satisfying!

If you eat bland or the same type of menu over & over what will happen psychologically, you'll get bored and start to reach for the unhealthy burger or Hot dog stand then your healthy eating plan goes straight out of the window!

Keep in your pantry a good stock of variety of healthy foods and ingredients e.g., variety of spices, vegetables, fruits, salads, wheat germ, wholefoods etc as the saying goes Variety is the Spice of Life!

Do colourful dishes too the more the variety of colour the better it is for you!

By having variety will keep your diets interested and not let you go off course!

The more colours there are the more the variety of vitamins and minerals your consuming!

For an example try a variety of salads mix & match with peppers reds, greens, yellows, toss in some tuna bites or add some protein e.g., slices of chicken breast or lean turkey slices, or hard-boiled eggs sliced with your salads!

Experiment with different dishes there are so many healthy dishes which are good for you to choose from. If you're stuck for some ideas to start your brand-new eating makeover just google 'healthy low-fat recipes' just see how many will come up on google!

Tip 4: Don't always finish your Plate!

Only eat as much as you feel comfortable without finishing everything on the plate! Don't feel guilty about it, be proud of yourself for Not overeating!

Also, a solution to this and to save waste, is to do smaller portions beforehand or use smaller plates!

Tip 5: Planning & Preparedness

Plan your Meals ahead of time.

Find time to sift through the many healthy recipes you have to hand from your collection of healthy meals, meal recipes, your healthy recipes sources and google!

If you plan your healthy mealtimes, you can avoid last minute unhealthy food choices!

Tip 6: Get Enough Sleep

Try to get a least 6-7 or even 8 hours of sleep a night!

It is well known tiredness is a key cause of emotional overeating! Studies show there is a big connection between lack of sleep and being overweight.

Tip 7: To Avoid being Hungry on Your Healthy Journey

To avoid being hungry on your new healthy schedule try to split up your calories into smaller meals. Say you're on 1500 calories a day, break them down into 5 or 6 small meals and you will avoid being hungry and be getting the recommended calories without overindulging.

Tip 8: Do remember their will always be Setbacks in a weight loss schedule.

Some days your body may retain water or your metabolism may be a bit slower that day.

Just stick to your planned healthy schedule and your goals of losing weight and being healthier will be fulfilled without you realising it!

Tip 9: Being Consciously Aware

Being consciously aware or another name for it is Mindfulness of what you are eating. For many people eating just becomes a habit an unconscious activity.

People meet up with their friends have drinks & decide to have all the same without realising that large calorie meal is contributing to weight gain and they eat the same to be sociable and not to make things awkward, also you can be distracted by watching TV or chatting on your phone it's so easy to wolf down the food without thinking about it!

Try to be more **mindful** take the time to focus on the pleasure of what you're eating, its presentation the texture, the smell and taste.

It will make you feel happier you've chosen to stick with healthier satisfying delicious food.

Tip 10: Carry A Notebook

If possible, when food shopping carry a notebook to record the best Low calorie/Low sugar products. Look out for the healthier alternatives.

All food products now should have the food contents ingredients and the red labels on the front of packages/tins stating the sugar, fats, saturated fats, calories, added ingredients etc.

This is now by law and give the consumer the choice whether to purchase the item or not.

Also, for **Tip 10** keep another Notebook with you to record everything and I mean everything you eat.

By doing this you can see for yourself just how many calories you're consuming, and it will show you a snapshot of your new healthy eating regime; by keeping all the great healthy recipes you discovered along the way.

You'll immediately see the new recipes you've created to the old type of foods you were eating previously.

Tip 11: Fruit & Fibre

Don't forget to add more fresh fruit, Fibre, and Vegetables to your regular diet! Today there is so much variety of new fruits and vegetables to choose from, just give them a try!

Tip 12: Food Colours

Make mealtimes as Fun as possible too in your dishes it's true the more colours there are the more the variety of vitamins & minerals, you're / consuming.

Tip 13: Two Words
Determination   Self-Discipline

Tip 14: Relaxation

Don't forget to make time for relaxation, to combat stress

Tip 15: Keep Hydrated
Don't forget to drink Water throughout the day! Regular fresh water drinking throughout the day, decrease your risk of dehydration plus helps rid body of excess toxins

Tip 16: Portion Sizes

Healthy foods too can be high in calories, so do keep an eye on portion sizes.

Don't forget to drink Water
throughout the day every day!'

If you want to get healthy again and lose weight too you can do it!

Keep to your schedule with Self-discipline and determination and you'll be amazed at the results you'll see in a short time.

Your goal will be a much healthier body and a much more positive outlook on life for your future happiness.

Some Healthy Sample Breakfasts to Try

Day 1

- 1 bowl of Muesli with soy milk
- 1 Glass of Orange Juice
- 1 cup of Tea

Day 2

- Poached eggs on spinach with garlic dressing
- 1 cup of decaffeinated coffee
- 1 glass of water

Day 3

- Bowl of Porridge Oats
- 1 glass of apple juice
- 1 cup of Tea

If you'd like a smoothie for breakfast which are healthy,
I've included some healthy smoothie recipes below for you to try, there are some healthy fruit shakes to consider for breakfast as an alternative

Banana Berry Shake

- ½ banana cut in chunks
- ½ pear cored & sliced
- Mixed fruit berries from frozen
- Low fat orange juice half a cup
- Low fat yogurt 1/3 of a tub
- Pour in blender thoroughly mix in and serve

- Mixed Fruit Eclipse

- 1 mandarin orange
- 1 Banana
- Half pack mixed frozen fruit
- Orange juice Low fat plain yogurt
- Pour in blender thoroughly mix in and serve

CHAPTER 5

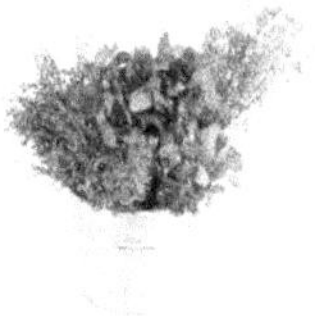

Some Low-Calorie Dishes For you to Try with Less than 300 Calories

Turkey or Chicken and Vegetable Curry

- Serves 4 * reduce recipe amount for less people/servings
- Preparation time: 30 mins Cook 40-45 mins Calories per portion 245 approx.
- A Delicious Easy to Make Curry that won't make you pile on the pounds and within your new diet schedule

- Sliced Turkey Slices or Chicken Breasts thawed chopped and diced

- 2 tablespoon vegetable or Sunflower Oil
- 1 Onion (adjust for extra people)
- 2 Cloves garlic crushed
- 1 tablespoon/5ml Chilli powder
- 1 tablespoon/5ml ground Coriander
- 1 tablespoon/5ml ground Cumin
- 1 tablespoon/5ml ground Turmeric
- 1 Potato peeled and diced (adjust for extra people)
- 2 Carrots peeled and diced (adjust for extra people)
- 1 Parsnip peeled and diced (adjust for extra people)
- 1 Can chopped tomatoes
- 1 Pint Chicken Stock
- Cauliflower Florets (adjust for extra people)
- 1 tablespoon/5ml Cornflower
- 1tablespoon/15ml Chopped Fresh Coriander

Method:

- Heat the Oil in a pan, add the onions and garlic and cook for 3 mins drain and put aside

- Cook the diced Turkey or Chicken (either) fry meat until browned all over.
- Stir in all the spices and a pinch of salt* optional and black pepper cook until browned and tender.
- Add the part cooked potatoes, carrots, and parsnip.
- Fry altogether until softening, pour in chopped tomatoes and stock and bring all to the boil. Toss in the cauliflower florets reduce heat and simmer for about 30 mins.
- Mix cornflower well in 2 tablespoon/30ml water add to curry simmer for 3 mins until thickened.
- Remove the pan from the heat and stir in chopped coriander.
- Can adjust seasonings to taste and serve curry with rice, plus optional poppadum, onion barges, vegetable samosas.

Remember though those extras do carry more calories to beware of.

For a lighter meal:

Tagliatelle with Peppers:

Made with crunchy Red & Green Yellow peppers and Aubergine

A Healthy Pasta Supper Dish Serves 6 * reduce recipe amount for less people

- Preparation time: 20 mins
- Cook time: 20 mins
- Calories per portion: 235 * adjust recipe amounts for extra people

-
- 1 Large Aubergine Sliced and Diced
- 1 Red Pepper 1 Green Pepper 1 Yellow Pepper sliced deseeded
- Pinch of Salt plus black pepper (optional)
- 12 to 14 oz Tagliatelle
- 1 tablespoon/15 ml Olive Oil or Vegetable Oil
- 1 tablespoon/15 ml Chopped Basil
- Sprigs of Basil to garnish optional
- Freshly grated low fat parmesan cheese
- Low fat vegetarian sausages can cut up into bite size portions

Method:

- Heat the Oil in a pan, add the Diced Aubergines cook until tender
- Cook the peppers in the oil until tender toss in the cooked aubergines. Drain into another dish for now leave to cool.
- Cook the Tagliatelle according to the instructions and until al dente
- Cook the vegetarian sausages and cut up into bite size pieces, adjust sausages to how many calories you wish to save
- Drain the pasta and add all the peppers, bite size sausages altogether mix and sprinkle with parmesan cheese arrange on serving plates.
- For extras can add some cherry tomatoes on a side dish optional

For a Summer or Winter Meal Low Calorie: Low fat vegetarian

A Healthy Roast Supper Dish Serves 2 * Add more recipe amount for more people

-	Preparation time: approx. 20 mins
-	Cook time: 25 mins
-	Calories per portion: 235 * adjust recipe amounts for extra people

Cheese & Vegetable Roast: By Anna Wing*

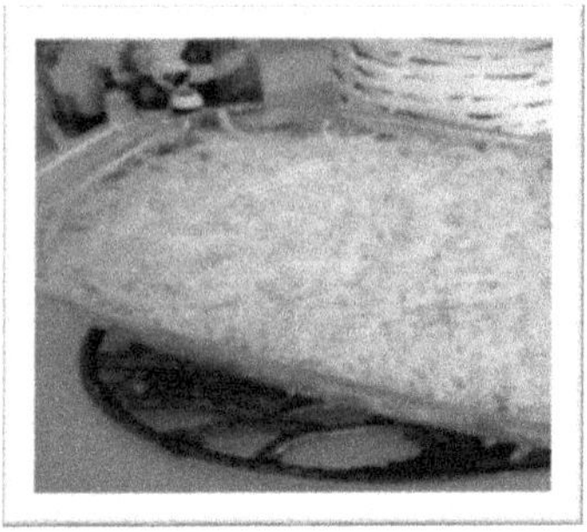

- 12 oz Mushrooms
- 1 Red Pepper 1 Green Pepper sliced deseeded
- 1 Onion Pinch of Salt plus black pepper (optional
- 3 tablespoon/15 ml Olive Oil or Vegetable Oil
- 3 Celery Sticks
- 8ozWholemeal breadcrumbs or plain

- 6oz Cheddar Low Fat Cheese
- Freshly grated low fat parmesan cheese
- 1 large Egg Salt & black pepper to taste

Method:

- Heat the Oil in a pan, Cook the peppers in the oil until tender
- Add the mushrooms and part cooked Celery cook until tender
- Remove from heat & stir in 6oz breadcrumbs & 4oz cheese adjust ingredients for more people
- Beat egg and add seasoning add to pan mixing everything together
- Spoon into baking dish smooth surface of dish
- Mix in the remaining cheese and breadcrumbs and sprinkle on top over the dish
- Cook for approx. 25 mins till brown can serve with extras Salad and garlic bread optional

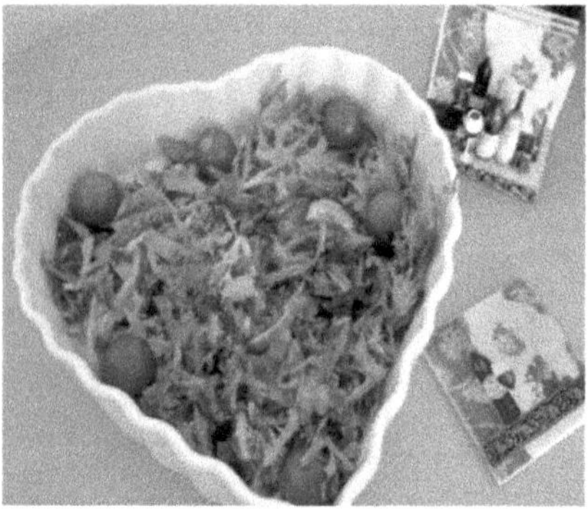

Spicy Bean Burgers:

For a Summer Outdoor Treat Low Calorie Meal:
- Calories per portion: 202 * adjust recipe amounts for extra people - Low fat vegetarian: - Preparation time: approx. 10 mins - Cook time varies 4-5 mins on pan - Makes 4 Burgers Adjust amounts for more servings

- 1 Can 14oz Cannellini Beans rinsed & drained
- 2 tablespoons Red Pesto
- ½cupWholemeal breadcrumbs
- 1 Large Egg
- 4 Spring Onions chopped & trimmed
- 1 garlic clove peeled & crush
- Pinch salt & fresh ground pepper
- 4 teaspoon sunflower oil (1 tsp per burger)

Method:

- Crush or mash up the beans. Add in the pesto, breadcrumbs, egg, onions & crushed garlic
- Pinch salt & pepper mix up well.
- Divide the mixture into 4 portions & form into balls. Place on a baking tray. Flatten the ball down with palm to form a burger shape.
- For best results chill the burgers 20 mins to help retain their shape.
- When you are ready to cook the burgers:
- Heat the oil over medium heat, add the burgers to pan and cook for about 4-5 mins on each side until golden.
- Serve hot with courgettes, or salad optional

For a Summer or Winter Meal Low Calorie:
Low fat vegetarian

A Healthy Med Spiced Chilli Dish Serves 2 Preparation time: approx. 15 mins Cook time: 25 mins Calories per portion: 220 * adjust recipe amounts for extra people

Soya made Chilli Con Carne:

- 3 tablespoon/15 ml Olive Oil or Vegetable Oil
- 1 Red Pepper 1 Green Pepper sliced deseeded
- 1 Onion Pinch of Salt plus ground black pepper (optional)
- 12 oz Mushrooms (optional)
- 1 Tin Chopped Tomatoes
- Tin 400 g Kidney Beans or Cannelloni mixed beans rinse and drained
- 8 oz Savoury Soya Protein Mince (cook this first in water on hob 4 mins)
- Pinch Salt*(optional) & black ground pepper to taste

Method:

- Heat the Oil in a pan, Cook the peppers and the Onion in the oil until tender Drain the peppers of oil in sieve return to pan. Cook the mushrooms (optional) mix
- Add 1 tin Chopped tomatoes Add the part cooked Soya mince mix all the ingredients together in pan
- Bring to the boil and simmer for 15 minutes or until thickened.
- Serve on a bed of cooked savoury rice (wholemeal garlic bread optional)
- Serves 2-3 * adjust recipe amounts for extra people

Low Calorie Dessert's

- Serves 6 **reduce recipe amount for less people
- Preparation time: 20 mins Cook 20 mins Calories per portion 235
- *(adjust recipe amounts for extra people)

Low Calorie Dessert

Apple & Fig or Sultana Crumble

- 5 oz. wholemeal plain Flour
- 2 Oz Brown sugar to taste
- 20z Low fat olive spread margarine
- 1lb Cooking Apples or Rhubarb
- Dried Figs or 8oz Sultanas
- Rind of lemon and juice of lemon
- Ground cinnamon 1bsp

Method:

- Sift flour into a large bowl, add the low-fat spread and lightly rub in with fingertips until the mixture resemble breadcrumbs stir in brown or demerara sugar.

- Place the partly cooked fruit into a 2-pint ovenproof dish, add the washed sultana's lemon juice and cinnamon.
- Spoon the crumble mix over the fruit and bake gas mark 4 20 mins or until golden brown.
- Serve hot or cold.

Mango & Lychee mousse

- Serves 8 **reduce recipe amount for less people
- Preparation time: 5 mins Plus Chilling time Calories per portion 84

- 400g can mango slices in juice
- 13 oz. can of lychees
- 2 tbsp. low-fat natural yogurt
- 4 tbsp. fromage frais
- 1 tsp lime juice
- 1 tbsp. skimmed-milk powder
- ½ tsp vanilla essence
- 2 tsp clear honey
- Rind from orange and lime to decorate

Method:

Place all ingredients except the rind in a blender or food processor blend altogether
For a thicker consistency add 1 extra tbsp. of skimmed milk powder Divide the mixture among 8 dessert (or less) glasses and chill for at least 30 minutes Decorate with a little pared orange and lime rind

For a Healthy Shake any time-of-day Blackberry Smoothie

Makes about 2 cups

- 1 cup (4oz/125 g) fresh or thawed frozen blackberries
- 1 cup (8 fl oz/250ml) milk
- ½ cup (4oz/125g) plain (natural) or mixed berry yogurt
- 1 teaspoon finely grated orange zest
- Place all ingredients in a blender and process until smooth and frothy
- Serves 2 (16 Fl oz /500 ml)

Mango and ginger lassi

This lassi makes a refreshing dessert following a curry.

- 1 large mango, peeled and flesh cut from pit
- 1 cup (8 oz/250g) plain (natural) yogurt
- ½ inch (12mm) piece fresh ginger peeled and chopped
- ½ cup (4 fl oz/125 ml) water, chilled
- 8 ice cubes (optional)
- 2 teaspoons sugar or to taste (optional)
- Place all ingredients in a blender and process until smooth.
- Taste and adjust or omit sugar to your liking.
- Makes about 2 ½ cups serves 2 or 3 adjust ingredients for more people.

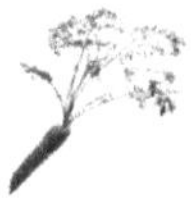

These are just a snapshot of some foods to do you good and have an anti-inflammatory property and there are probably a lot more……

Top 20 Anti-inflammatory foods:

- Apples
- Cherries
- Carrots
- Nuts
- Onions
- Courgettes
- Aubergines
- Green Leafy Vegetables (kale, spinach, broccoli)
- Oily Fish like salmon, sardines, haddock
- Beans
- Turmeric
- Dark Chocolate
- Red/Peppers/Green
- Red kidney beans
- Tomatoes
- Peaches
- Olives
- Seeds such as chia seeds pumpkin, linseed
- Some fresh Yogurts
- Tea plus Green Tea

CHAPTER 6

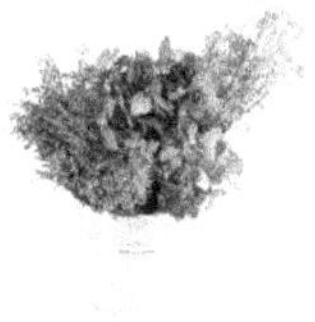

Exercise Routines & Stick to your Planning

Do you after your evening meal start to fall asleep or feel like you need a sleep?

Do you have a drowsy feeling you cannot shake off and stays with you throughout the day every day it feels like!

Remember this OTHER quote I am going to give you and try to memorise it each day!

'Inactivity causes tiredness' and tiredness is a side effect of Inactivity'.

If you can try to put this quote on your fridge door, somewhere where you can see it each day eventually you will remember it.

Any day your feeling tired 'or a bit down say the quote to yourself. 'Inactivity causes tiredness' and tiredness is a side effect of inactivity'.

Many people when they get to a certain age blame their 'tiredness' on their age!

They tell their Dr's I expect to feel this way 'it's my age' because I am old!

They feel they are in a circle and it is all part of life, get to an age, pile the weight on, get health problems and thus blame all this on 'my age', so give up and accept it without doing anything about it! But it does not have to be like this, yes were all getting old that's nature but you are getting old long before your time a lot sooner than you need to!

There are some elderly pensioners who are keeping fit some are still running the London Marathon, several time over too!

All you need to do is to be determined and just make a few adjustments in your life, by eating healthily, and becoming a lot more active you will be surprised what you can achieve and how your life can change.

By being more active like you were in your teens! there will be no going back!
If the idea of doing any fitness routine put's you off or makes you very nervous, or you have health issues/ mobility issues then you could start your new fitness routine with 'baby steps' and when you're feeling more confident and notice a difference, you'll automatically want to do more!

It has been well known that an aerobic type of exercise produces a powerful hormone called endorphins, the body makes more of this hormone during endurance type exercises.

Endorphins give you a 'feel good' feeling and a feeling of wellbeing. Plus, in some cases endorphins have been shown to be a powerful painkiller.

Today there are numerous exercise programs and start-up classes for overweight people and unfit beginners.

Most of these start-up classes assess you from the beginning, devise a beginners' program suitable for your needs and you can start at a comfortable pace that suits you.
You will build up your fitness through a gradual process and over time you will start to see the rewards.

What you will need though to take with you is a bit of patience, determination and lastly discipline to get you to where you really want to be.

Your never 'too old' or too unfit to make that change! There are some great advantages to getting fit too!

If you stick with an 'aerobic' type of fitness, you will gain a 'training effect' a superb side effect of your great effort to get fit!

The 'training effect' will see you have a have a new outlook on life, you will be able to tolerate stress better and sleep better too! As well as looking good!

We're going to get you fit! By getting your fitness training up to scratch or attempting to get more activity (aerobic) if possible, in your life you will start to notice a difference and how that 'tiredness' will begin to disappear!

You will have more 'oxygen' rich energy, have a better outlook on life, and will want to do livelier and more energetic things.

There are many Aerobic /cardio activities you can incorporate into your life;

it doesn't have to be an all-out unplanned rushed exhausting slog as doing it that way won't work for you and you're likely want to give up before you've even started.

Did you know by just walking is an aerobic activity? Find an aerobic activity you enjoy the most one you feel most comfortable with which you enjoy that way you'll stick with it and keep yourself motivated. Over time you will see great results.

Added bonus you'll lose weight without even thinking about it You'll be having fun reaching your goals and will keep motivated if you enjoy the chosen activity and not pushing yourself too hard!

CHAPTER 7

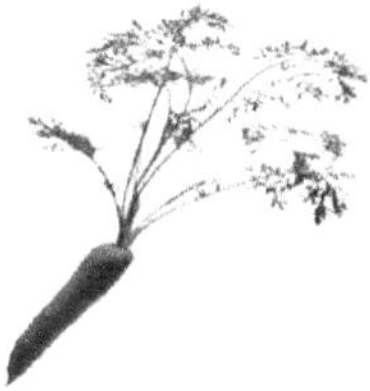

The Benefits of Cardio Exercise

- Stronger heart
- Your heart will not have to work as hard to pump your blood
- Lung Capacity Greatly Increased
- Burns Fat and Calories for weight loss without you even noticing
- Will reduce your risk of: A heart attack, high blood pressure, Diabetes, high cholesterol,
- Makes you feel good: Relieves depression, reduces stress, relieves anxiety
- Helps you sleep better
- Improves sex life
- Builds stronger muscles especially in your legs
- Gives you more confidence, self-esteem, makes you feel happier

- To get the benefits of cardio you don't have to do hours of high impact cardio.

You can benefit from a 10–15-minute walk in the fresh air.

You can with time build up longer cardio time as you progress but always do what feels comfortable and build up gradually.

Ideally keep a workout diary to record your progress by keeping a diary you will see how much you've improved and progressed.

Start out slowly each day and take rest days in between.

For anyone with health problems or severely overweight and has not exercised in a long time do take your Drs/physicians advice first.

Cardio for Severely Overweight or Obese People:

Firstly, **get checked out from your doctor take his/her** advice that its ok to start any aerobic program.

If you are a bit daunted or feel nervous about starting a cardio program because you have not exercised for an exceptionally long time, try to begin doing a sitting aerobic program.

There are now numerous new innovative cycle machines on the market which you can pedal whilst you are sitting down, this would be a great starter as you would still be stimulating your joints and improving your circulation.

These pedal cycles are great for people who currently have difficulty getting around or feel nervous starting out too fast starting an aerobic type of exercise.

You can gradually each day increase the repetitions (try to keep a record) you can go at your own pace and stop anytime if you have any kind of discomfort.

By keeping a record, you will be able to see your results.

Try to be consistent positive and do not give up.

I would say if you can manage it to start do 5-8 mins each day on the pedal machine

Gradually increase the minutes either daily or weekly whichever suits you better

If you've kept to the schedule and feel that you've improved over the weeks you could after time upgrade your pedal cycle for an exercise bike.

Again, starting off slowly, only progressing when you feel comfortable on the bike then maybe increasing the duration over time.

It is not a rush do what you feel comfortable with and always listen to your body.

Also, there are some great walking programs for beginners online which can take you through your paces from very beginners to more advanced programs.

Do check them out if you have a PC or Laptop with speakers, the programs are very motivating as your working out at the same time with others!

Take rest days in between exercise this gives your muscles a rest and time for muscles and body to rebound and adjust to the demands placed upon it.

As your body fitness starts to improve you will find subtle changes too to your eating habits your appetite may change, you may find sometimes your less hungry and your desires for unhealthy foods

e.g., sweet things, bad carbs, and fast foods etc you will find yourself searching for more healthier options, this is a great side effect for getting fitter.

CHAPTER 8

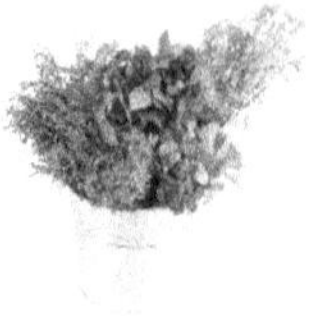

Stress and how to deal with it

Today we are more stressed than ever before! And outside sources like Brexit, Employment worries, pandemic cost of living worries, etc etc.......

it just adds more and more fear for us and it is no wonder were so stressed!

It is also affecting our children they see their parents stressed and they are picking it up themselves plus they are seeing or hearing news bulletins which frightens them even more!

Young children should not have a care in the world but they are inheriting this stress from things around them!

In the past no one had even heard of the word Anxiety and Stress but now it is spoken of daily of someone being stressed about something, and now we have so many disorders related to stress!

- Depression
- Panic Attacks
- Anxiety Disorder
- OCD
- Social Anxiety
- Anorexia

The list goes on but what can we do about it?

We get over one crisis then round the corner another crisis hits us just as we were getting back on our feet.
Today it seems like everyone we meet is on some type of medication to help relieve their stress and cope with life.

It not only affects us mentally it affects us physically too! Heart attacks, cancer, IBS, high blood pressure …………
If we could wave a magic wand and stop being stressed that would be great!

But we just don't have an antidote.

We must try to stop people being so stressed and seeing a loved one get ill but as we are human beings, we are always going to experience stressful situations.

We cannot escape the unfortunate bad events that we have no power over, the things which hit us really hard!

Such as bereavement, loss of a job, a home, bad news etc….

We are all going to have to deal with stress in our lives so it is better to know how to react to stress in a positive way so that we can control our behaviour and not allow stress to become a health threat.

What is Stress?

Stress is when a different or unexpected event occurs to our usual peaceful routine.

It throws us off balance, takes us by surprise and makes us fearful which in turn makes us stressed!

It is the same for our children if something changes ….

for example, the parents get a divorce, this would be frightening for them as their world as they know it has been turned upside down and through their fears lead to them experiencing anxiety and stress!

Stress is a bad event that happens to us out of the blue which disrupts our once peaceful and calm life.

Also, apart from bad news and bad events we have to try to recognise the things making us so frightened that it's affecting our daily lives!

But How Can We Deal With It?

We must try to:

- Identify before it happens the stressors that affect us
- Try to eliminate or avoid the things we know will upset us

- Learn how we can manage our stress and pass on this knowledge to our children
- Use an outside source (if things get so bad) to help us to learn and train ourselves to relax

Some people are driven or overworked, when they come home from work or even at weekends, they still feel super hyped!

- They really struggle to wind down and relax this can happen to shift workers too!

But to keep this up constantly wears the body down and eventually this is where 'Stress' sets in!

To be constantly 'wound up' after say working in a high-powered job or a career that keeps a person working 35-60 hr week and shift workers included it is really hard to 'switch off'

Many people in this category just cannot relax and may have to take training or seek out some sort of outside source to help them to learn to relax!

Fortunately, there is an answer to this problem.

There is an antidote if that person will just take it upon themselves to learn to live more calmly/serenely in this age of anxiety and stress!

If you are experiencing this type of constant stress, I am going to mention even advise you to practice two powerful training methods, I say 'training' because it's gone beyond knowing how to do it yourself:

- Deep/breathing techniques
- Yoga/relaxation techniques.

These two if practised on a regular basis will certainly complement each other and will help you and teach you how to relax both your mind and body.
But you say how and where do I find the time?

I will be honest you have to make and find the time because if you continue and do nothing and continue with your stressful lifestyle...

You will welcome in serious illness which in turn will affect not only your job/career but also your family life too.

There are numerous resources out there to help you.

Publications/books, classes to attend in your neighbourhood or private establishments but you must make that effort yourself if you want to change your life around.

CHAPTER 9

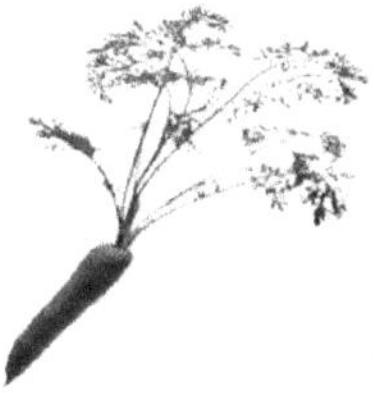

Relaxation

Remember this quote:

'There can be No Physical relaxation without the mental.'

No Mental relaxation without the Physical'

This is how entwined our mental fitness has an effect on our physical fitness and vice versa.

Many people with boring, easy routine, jobs have expressed 'I haven't done a thing all day but feel 'dead tired.'

This is a body which has not done much all day but is eating oneself up with Tension!

It is the speed and strains of modern life, modern technology, and the extremely fast tempo at which we live.

Pressure, noise, deadlines, news bulletins, tv, etc…. we cannot escape.

Consider how much better you will feel after a few minutes of Deep Relaxation. To escape for just a few minutes the hustle & bustle. To close yourself off from everything and relax.

If you learn these techniques especially during yoga practice alone at home or in a group you will learn to 'let go.' Your muscles will relax and your mind will relax.

You are ridding your body and mind of all tension for a few minutes. Imagine if you did this on a regular schedule how you will start to feel.

To learn to relax completely especially if you have been constantly stressed and, on the go, **will take practice.**

You will not be able to master it in one lesson but if you're willing to try and take up the lessons you'll be helping yourself and getting the life back you deserve!

With regular Deep Relaxation practice and proper Deep Breathing practice combined with yoga practice you will certainly learn to manage stress better!

I will give you some practice techniques on both relaxation and deep breathing these are only practices but if you have any health issues or any concerns before practicing do, please take advice from your doctor first:

Deep Relaxation practice

Do you find after a busy stressful day at work or you've just been nonstop in some other pastime Just busy, busy; and you find when it comes to bedtime you just cannot let go and relax?

Your adrenaline is still pumping and you just feel this is going to be another sleepless night? Only to wake up exhausted for another day ahead.

There is an antidote to this dilemma but it will take patience and practice and eventually you will be able to do it naturally again and again once you have learnt the technique.

You will learn **to let go as many muscles as possible** and as many thoughts as possible.

To do this your brain and body will rest to the very core of your being and in Yoga practice this relaxation technique is called the Death pose or another word being used is The Sponge.

Meaning your body would be so relaxed it can soak anything up and you would not worry.

The object of this exercise is to rid your body of all conscious tension and muscles of contraction so that you are resting every fibre of your body.

Because you are constantly on the go your causing more and more tension to build up and you are not taking time out to relax or give your body and mind some respite.

Basically, you are giving yourself more and more tension, and tension is the enemy of all achievement!

Some people it is known are scared to relax they think if they do nothing and take time out everything will fall apart and they feel guilty for doing nothing because maybe they had it drilled into them from an early age that to progress in life you can't just let things go by doing nothing!
Resting on their laurels! Time is money etc.... so, they constantly feel the need to reach the deadline

whatever it takes! But you would probably reach your goal a lot quicker if you took some time out!

Below is the technique to practice the death pose or sponge. Give it a go but hopefully you will join a yoga

class where you will be able to learn the techniques one to one with your yoga teacher.

Sponge or Death Pose

- Promotes deep muscular relaxation
- Deeply relaxes nervous system
- Lie on the floor either on a yoga mat or carpet just so you feel comfortable Keep your legs flat and slightly apart arms floppy by your side.
- Once you feel settled take a couple of (Diaphragm) breaths then relax.
- Next point your toes forward away from you hold for 5 seconds relax
- If you feel any tension anywhere in your body, try to trace it, go through each muscle one by one to release the tension -- pretend you have swallowed a dissolvable magnetic tracer whose job is to pick up any nervous tension through each of your limbs—
- The magnetic tracer will start from your foot moving over each of your limbs until your whole body has been scanned by the tracer.

- ➢ It will help if you Follow the magnetic trace up through the legs, trunk, and arms where there is any trace of tension. Include the jaw, mouth, and face.
- ➢ Let your mind relax by thinking of nothing except the relaxation the magnetic tracer is working for you picking up all these tense nerves on the way.
- ➢ It will take practice to let go and feel really relaxed but you will master it better each time.
- ➢ Completely relax for about 2-5 minutes or when you feel like getting back up sometimes 5 minutes are enough it really depends how stressed you have felt and your body will tell you

The sponge is called Death Pose in Hindu Sanskrit.

This pose really is a Deep Relaxation where your body can be at complete rest.

Practicing this pose is an antidote for constantly being on the go and having or finding no time to relax.

After some weeks of practicing the sponge, you will be able to relax without having to go through the sequences and trying too hard it will come naturally!

Meditation

In this short description I will give a brief or a short insight to meditation and how it can benefit you particularly in conjunction with your yoga practice.

Also, you will learn more about meditation if you do decide to take up yoga and your yoga instructor will teach you meditation techniques so that you get a better understanding and will practice correctly.

Meditation

What is it and why should we practice it

Meditation is a practice in which an individual uses a technique – such as mindfulness or focusing the mind on a particular object, thought, or activity – to train for awareness and concentration; also, to achieve a mentally clear and emotionally calm and stable state.

It is a turning inward of one's senses and thoughts so that nothing from the outside world is experienced with a sense of complete relaxation and a feeling of great calm and contentment with the world. To understand and practice meditation correctly you will learn deep concentration first like concentrating on an object like a candle to the exclusion of everything else.

If you practice yoga your teacher will give you the option if you would like to learn meditation too.

CHAPTER 10

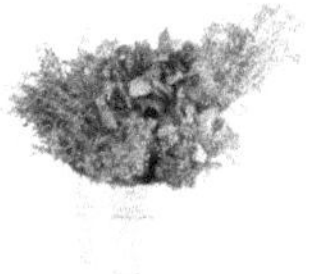

Deep Breathing

Below for you to take note of I have included a small piece of scientific fact on Deep Breathing

- The fact is very few of us breathe properly.
- If you look around you, you will be amazed the amount of people breathe through the mouth instead of through the nose.
- They inhale directly through the larynx allowing air to reach the bronchioles without it being properly warmed and filtered.

Air to be cleansed of bacteria & dust should be drawn through the nasal passages where the mucosa with secretions filters it.

- Also breathing through the nose allows the air which travels further is warmed to body temperature instead of hitting the lungs freezing cold which could cause the airways to constrict, plus mouth breathing can cause more colds and infections.

The best and proper way of breathing is done from the diaphragm

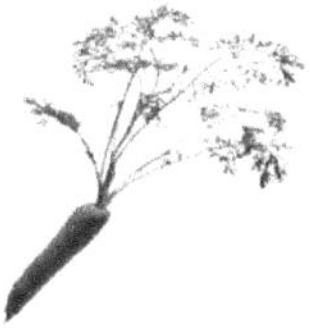

Health Benefits from Deep Breathing

- Anxiety
- Depression
- Improving Concentration/focus

- Better sleep
- Faster recovery from exercise
- Handling Stress better

- Blood Pressure reduces
- Pulse rate reduces

- Gives you a calming feeling
- Helps with your mental health by reducing stress
- When you take up yoga you will learn the correct way of breathing with many deep-breathing exercise techniques.

- With regular practice proper deep diaphragm breathing will come naturally and you will do it automatically.

Deep Breathing Practice

It is never too late to re-learn how to breathe correctly

– no matter your age. Especially if we are stressed

proper diaphragmatic breathing, is the key.

Try this practice method:

- Make yourself comfortable either by lying on your back or sitting.
- If sitting do, make sure you keep your back straight keep both feet on the floor. Release the tension in your shoulders by relaxing the shoulders.
- Close your eyes (by closing your eyes helps you to concentrate more on the exercise in hand rather than external stimuli.

Place one hand on your stomach and the other on your chest

- Take your normal breaths (how you normally breathe). Does your belly rise and fall with every breath in inhalation? And every breath out exhalation?
- If you answer 'yes' that is good. This is the natural way of breathing.

- If your belly stays still but your chest rises and falls with every breath you are shallow breathing and you will need to practice some diaphragmatic breathing.

- Continue to take deep breaths, but concentrating on only moving your belly, as you take a breath in through your nose, imagine a balloon being blown up in your stomach breathe out through your mouth as if you are blowing out through a straw.

- It can take some time relearning how to breathe correctly.
- With practice the easier it becomes.

- Do practice this exercise every day you can practice anywhere.

- The best time to practice this breathing is when you are relaxed. As you will take deeper breaths.

- If you can try to practice first thing in the morning and before you go to sleep. By practicing in the morning helps set the tone for the day and you will feel calmer and more relaxed.

- Same as for night practice this breathing it will prepare your mind and body for sleep.

- Eventually with time and practice you'll get an idea about how long you need to practice deep breathing exercises to help reduce stress. Practicing more often will help you master the deep breathing as it becomes a habit in your life.

- Do not give up. Diaphragmatic/deep breathing takes practice, and you may find it feels different if you're not used to breathing this way.

During times of extreme stress or panic or anxiety, deep breathing exercises can help you to feel calmer and more peaceful, after the unpleasant symptoms you've gone through.

Breathing exercises can help you

also, to work through hyperventilation which sometimes occur from overwhelming panic attacks and anxiety.

Deep breathing is a form of relaxation that will help you rid yourself of physical stress and mental strain.

There is another breath that (yogis)* (practicing) Yoga use in yoga practice it is called The 3 part-breath it is often used at the beginning of yoga practice.

I haven't given you this technique as it is best you practice this when and if you take up yoga practice;

I have given you one example the diaphragmatic breathing technique for you to practice if you wish.

Caution: As with all breathing exercises, do approach the practice with caution, especially if you have any health condition such as asthma, or any respiratory condition.

Stop any breathing exercise if you become dizzy or feel faint.
Always work with your fitness guide or yoga practitioner then you will never go wrong.

CHAPTER 11

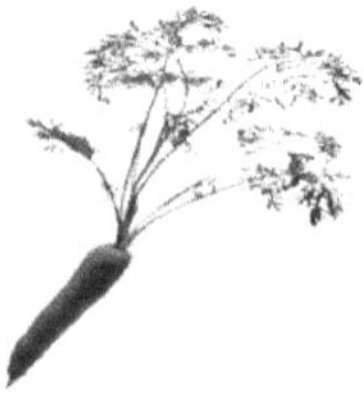

New Way of Working

If we did not breathe, we would not be able to survive and would die within minutes without oxygen.

The brain needs three times more oxygen than our other organs.

That is why people who have sedentary jobs almost always complain of 'tiredness' it's because they're not physically active enough, yes, they're working but using their brains to do the work.

It is well known sedentary workers are oxygen starved. They also are losing their fitness because of little movement in their working lives.

Now some companies have recognised this health issue and (at last) have started to think about the health of their workers.

Also, it could in effect cost the companies more money in staff sickness's due to the working conditions.
Enter the Treadmill Desk. And this trend is catching on not just with the manager's showing more care for their staff but the staff are more aware of this health issue and are liking their new workstation and are eager to take part!

There was a small study of 15 Obese Office workers where they were offered to walk and work on a moving treadmill workstation.
This was at a slow pace of 1 mile per hour!

They were monitored and the result was they burned an extra 100 calories per hour! They thus calculated if they used the Treadmill workstation for 2 to 3 hours daily, they estimated they could lose 44-66 pound per year!

In a 2013 study 36 subjects who used a treadmill desk for about 1 hour a day lost an average of 3.1 pounds, and the people who were Obese lost the most! Approx. 7.5 pounds an average of (3.4 kilograms).

Imagine if all companies adopted this practice gave a thought to their staff and set up these treadmill workstations, it would be an amazing feat in the real world!

It could transform more people's lives and could also help with putting an end to Obesity!

Just think about that, because being sedentary at work is one of the main reasons a cause of people becoming or prone to getting Obesity! and with all the health hazards that accompany it!

People now are becoming more aware of the dangers of being sedentary and sitting down all day!

And with all the publicity of this health hazard more people have decided to do something about it and are making changes to the way they live.

The sale of Treadmills for work or home use have risen exponentially these last few years and keeping fit on a treadmill or walking, running etc….

is now transforming people's lives and giving people a new purpose and optimism for their health, it is getting more and more people's lives fitter than they've been for years.

Not only by using exercise equipment like treadmills etc but now more and more people are using online exercise programs which feature on YouTube

There are walking programs, low impact aerobics programs, programs with other online people which give you the motivation as your working out together.

and by seeing other people doing the same thing really motivates you; you can also monitor your progress each day in the comfort of your home!

These online classes have really taken off.

CHAPTER 12

Tables To Keep

Below is a Table of Good Carbs List

These good foods I have given you are just a snapshot here there are hundreds of good carbs out there so do try to keep a record of these super foods and list all the new ones you find which will do you good.

Then you can say goodbye to bad eating food for good!

Good Carbs List

Vegetables	Fruit	Whole Grains
Acorn Squash	Apple	Buckwheat
Artichoke	Apricot	Millet
Asparagus	Banana	Oats
Aubergine	Blueberry	Quinoa
Beetroot	Coconut	Brown Rice
Broad Beans	Fig	Spelt
Broccoli	Mango	Sweet Potatoes
Brussel Sprouts	Papaya	Beets
Butternut Squash	Passion Fruit	Turnip
Cabbage	Peach	Avocado
Carrots	Pear	Oranges
Cauliflower	Plum	Zucchini
Celeriac	Lemon & Limes	Kale

Below is a Table of BAD Carbs List

White Bread	Ice Cream	Jams
Pastries	Most Cereals	Rich Desserts
Cakes/ Muffins	Energy Bars	Corn Crisps
Pies	Sausage Rolls	Croutons
White Rice	Fried Chips	Condensed Milk
Dressings	Pizza	Tortillas
Wines (sweet)	Pudding	Battered foods
Fizzy Drinks + Soda Pops	Biscuits (some)	Pork Pie
Candy	Pasta White	Pancakes (some).

Bad Carbs List Continued

Roast potatoes	Milk chocolate
jellies	Sweet yogurt
Barbecue sauce	bagels
Black pudding	White flour
Cola pop	waffles

These bad foods I have given you are just a snapshot there are hundreds out there so do be aware of the bad carbs and check the food out first how good or bad it is for you.

Bad Carbs:

- Feel hungry faster
- -Have added sugars preservatives, colorings, flavouring's etc.
- -Raised blood sugar quicker
- -Makes you fat easier and store it
- -High Glycaemic
- -Cannot burn many calories

It can be a minefield of not knowing what to eat so to put it into perspective I'm going to describe the basic differences of these good & bad carbs.

Bad carbohydrates have been altered and made refined.

Food manufacturers refined these carbs to make various products; to give example, whole wheat grain is refined to produce fine flour.

What occurs is the grains are stripped of Fibre, vitamins, minerals, and healthy fats which results in carbohydrates made refined and are stripped of valuable nutrients.

To add to these refined carbohydrates, have additives, preservatives, colourings, flavourings, added to them which is detrimental to our health!

Also, these refined carbs can impact blood sugar levels causing sudden rises and falls.

We do though need carbohydrates for our body to function. To give us energy, we have to be aware also that not all carbohydrates are bad for us.

Look out for the best carbs called Complex Carbohydrates which include good whole grains and a rich variety of vegetables there are so many new varieties of good food options to choose from out there!

I will give you another table to help you decide on better healthy food options the table is very similar to my Good Carbs Table.

It will help you too in your meal planning without getting stressed about knowing what is good or bad for you.

The Difference between Good Complex Carbs

Good Carbs:

- Keep you fuller for longer
- Natural sugars
- Does not raise blood sugar levels
- Take longer to Digest
- Great for Energy
- Low Glycaemic
- Help you lose Fat
- Easy Calorie Burns

Some Complex Carbs That Are Fine for Weight Loss Table:

Tomatoes	Wheat germ
Porridge	Shredded Wheat
Apples	Mueseli
Chia Seeds	Fruit & Vegetables
Pitta Breads	Whole wheat Pasta
Sweet Potatoes	Steel Cut Oats
Steel Cut Oats	Blueberries
Bananas	Zucchini
High fibre Cereals	Brown Rice
Chick Peas	Kidney Beans

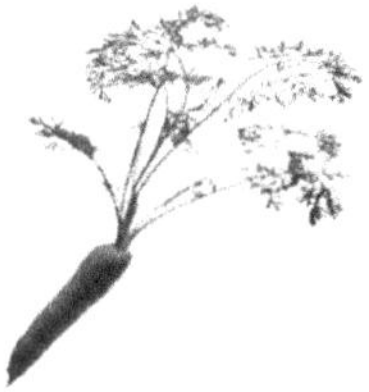

Your Diary and Progress

In this Chapter I have included for you a blank timetable below for you to fill in yourself, this will help you to choose your most favourite healthy meals, and it will be a record to keep of your favourite healthy foods/dishes.

You can refer to your timetable when stuck for ideas; at the same time, you can add to the list when you also source out for yourself new healthy recipes just add them to the timetable.

Soon you will have a huge catalogue of good healthy meals and dishes to choose from without you going off track and reaching for unsuitable fast foods!

Breakfast Lunch Dinner

Mon	Tues	Wed	Thurs	Frid	Sat	Sun
B						
L						
D						
B						
L						
D						
B						
L						
D						

My Healthy Complex Carbs Menu Weekly Timetable

You can if you wish create a table similar to keep an eye on your healthy lifestyle progress.

This Is completely optional but remember you're not going on a Diet just changing some things/behaviours in your life to feel better about yourself and a new healthier lifestyle

Week	Current Weight	Weight Loss
1		
2		
3		
4		
5		
6		
7		
8		
9		

Conclusion:

Some words from me to you

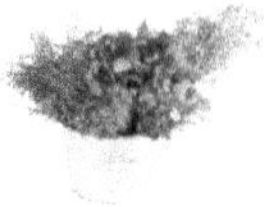

I hope I have given you some helpful and encouraging information and tips in my book.

If you follow some guidelines, I have included you will see a change and a new motivation to follow through.

It can be challenging today on how we can try to look after ourselves, the world is busy and hectic

And we forget to do things for ourselves we tend to cut corners.

But to keep healthy in mind and body we must make more time for ourselves and to be aware of the dangers that unhealthy living practices can do to us

Do Stay Motivated Stay Positive and thank you for reading.

Ingram Content Group UK Ltd.
Milton Keynes UK
UKHW022032290523
422506UK00015B/585

9 781739 103873